SIMPLIFIED HEART SOUNDS

Malcolm Rosenberg, R.N.

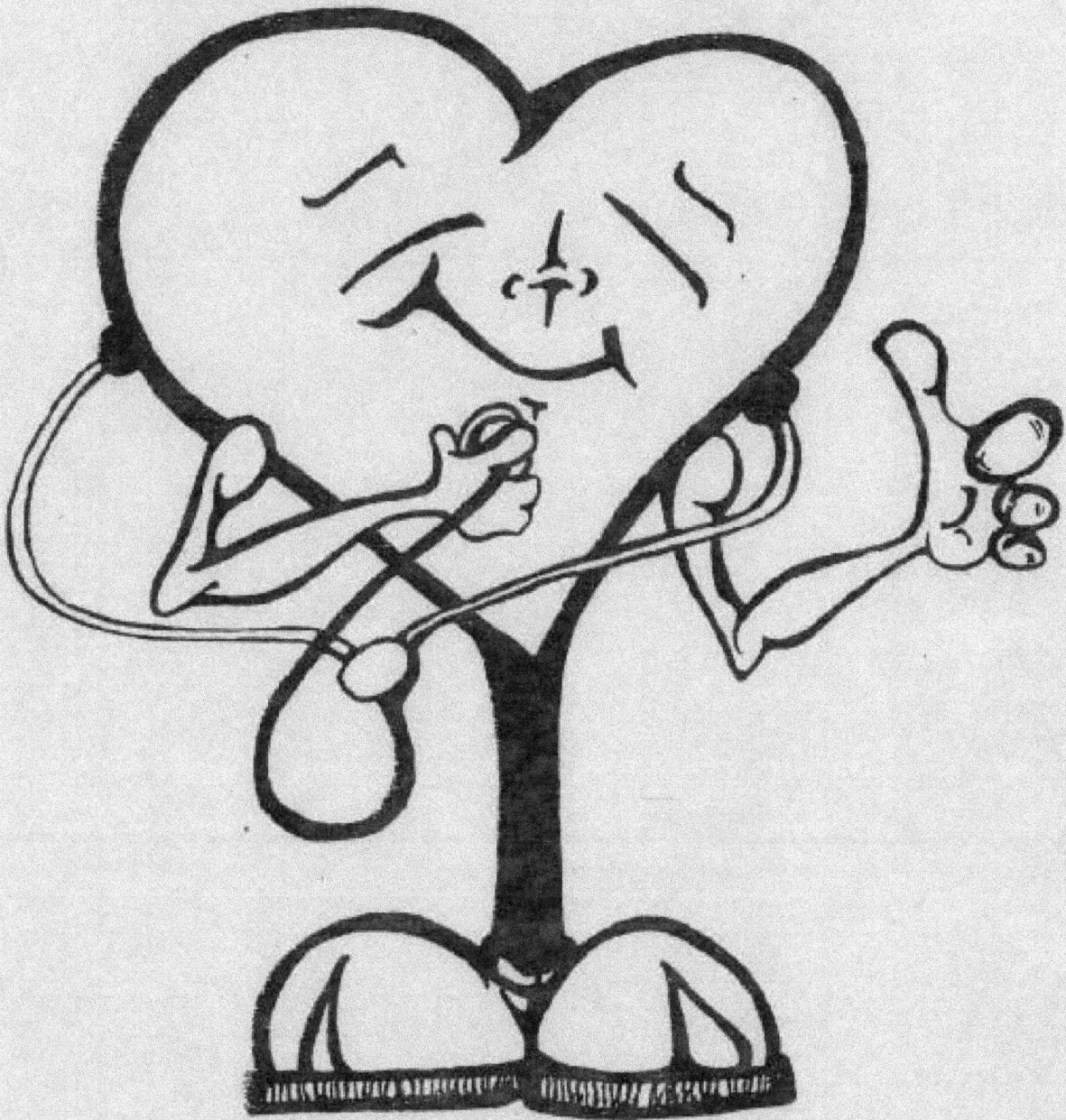

SIMPLIFIED HEART SOUNDS

Malcolm Rosenberg, R.N.

If you are watching an action thriller like Die Hard, and the hero is surrounded by the terrorists, you see shadows of their weapons then the camera turns to our sweat soaked, hopelessly outgunned hero Bruce Willis... and in the background Duh..dah...Duh..dah...Duh..dah.

That is Lesson One: Normal Heart Sounds. This pamphlet assumes you have seen Die Hard at least once. For those of you have seen it about twenty times, I assume you are reading this only to review normal heart sounds.

There are about 50 identifiable heart sounds that correlate to cardiac abnormalities and diseases. This pamphlet covers about 10.

As a nurse you are required only to know normal (Die Hard) heart sounds and to recognize anything abnormal. To pass hospital ICU tests these heart sounds are what you will need to know.

It would be better if an audio recording accompanied this pamphlet. If you want to pursue this subject there are books with recordings. In the mean time this is enough information to pass any test.

To stimulate your imagination, we will be using this diagram of the heart.

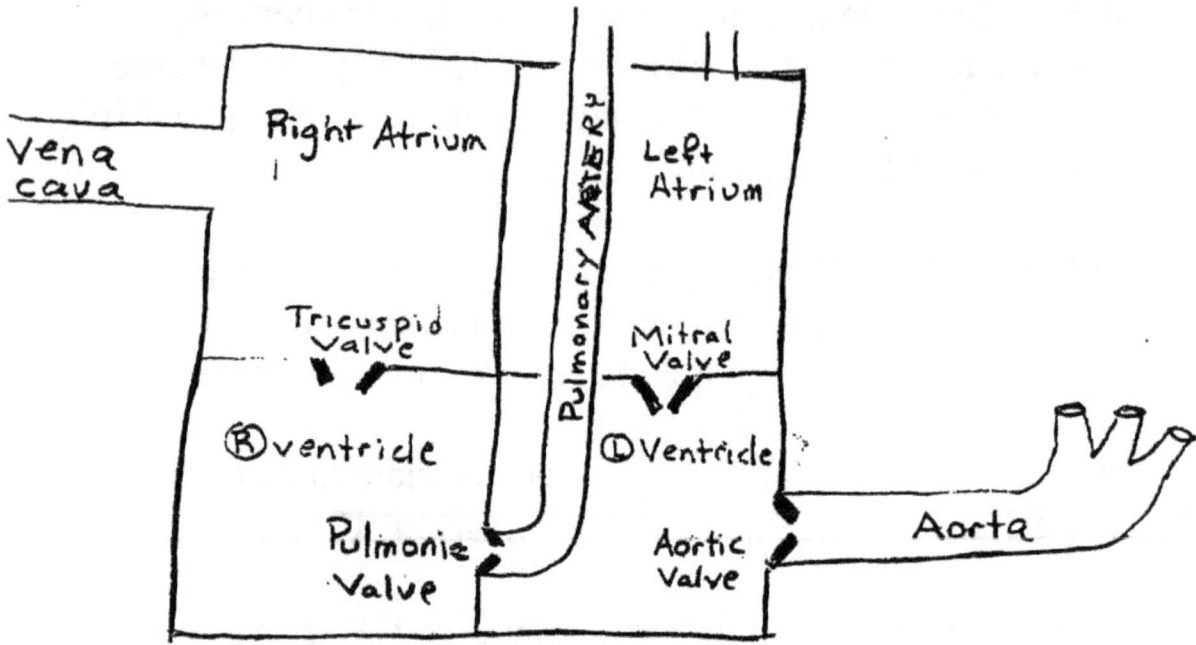

The four valves are shown as thick black lines.

Here they are shown open.

Here they are shown closed.

Light arrows surrounding the chambers show muscular contraction.

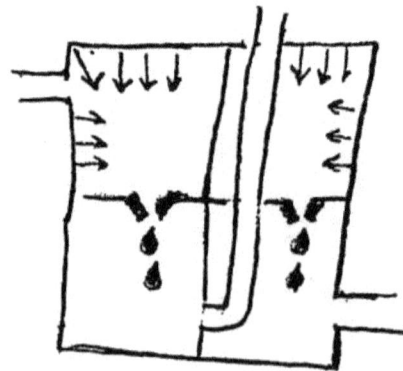

Blood flow is shown as drops.

Let's review a single heart beat.

The right atrium fills with deoxygenated blood from the vena cava and the left atrium fill with oxygenated blood from the pulmonary vein.

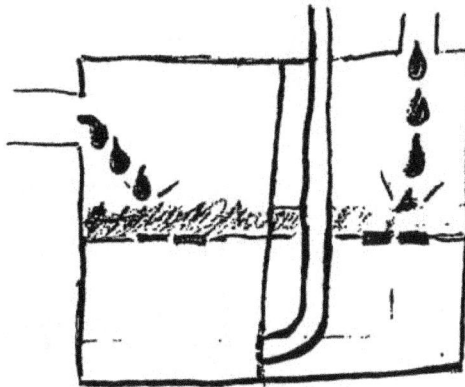

The mitral and tricuspid valves open due to low pressure in the ventricles.

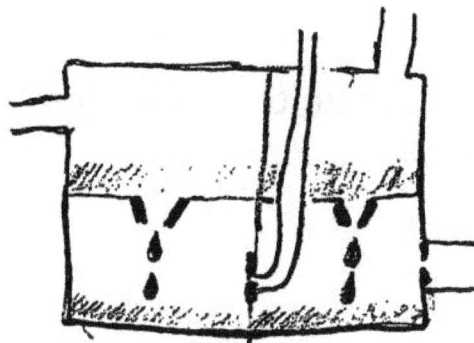

The sinus node initiates the electrical charge along the neural pathways that stimulate the atria to contract and squeeze out the rest of the blood to complete the filling of the ventricles.

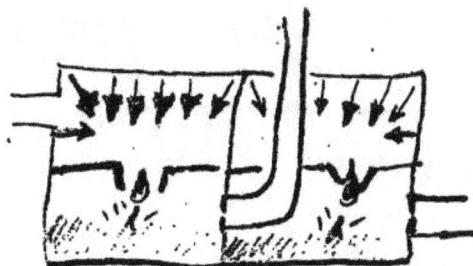

The electrical charge follows the pathway through the AV node to the ventricles where it causes forceful contraction. The high ventricular pressure closes the mitral and tricuspid valves and pushes open the aortic and pulmonic valves. Blood is squeezed into the lungs and the rest of the body.

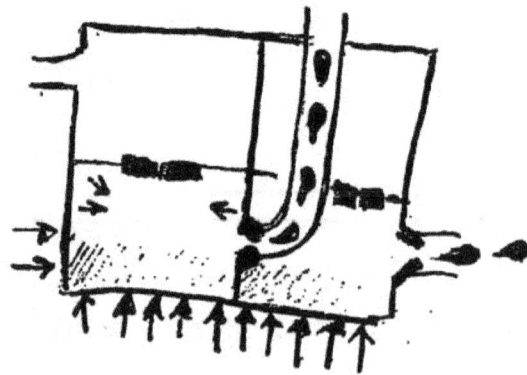

After the blood is squeezed out, the ventricles relax and the aortic and pulmonic valves snap shut.

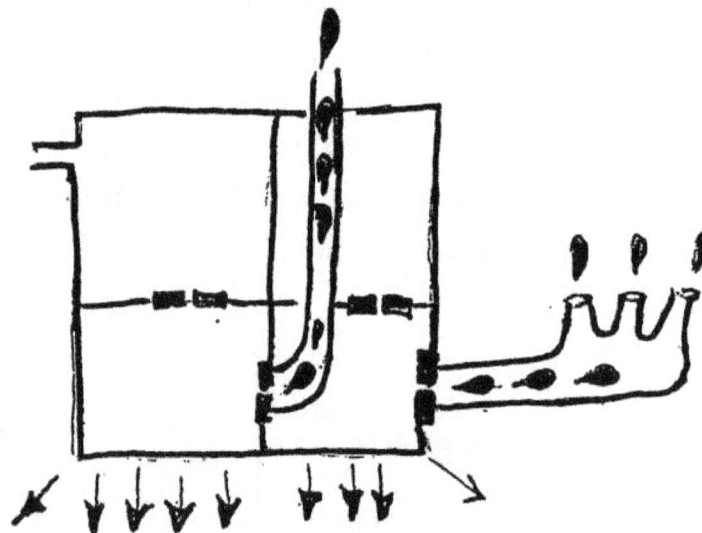

NORMAL HEART SOUNDS

S1 S2 "Lub Dub"

"Lub" The beginning of systole: after blood has been squeezed into the into the ventricles, the ventricles contract and the mitral and tricuspid valves snap shut. S1

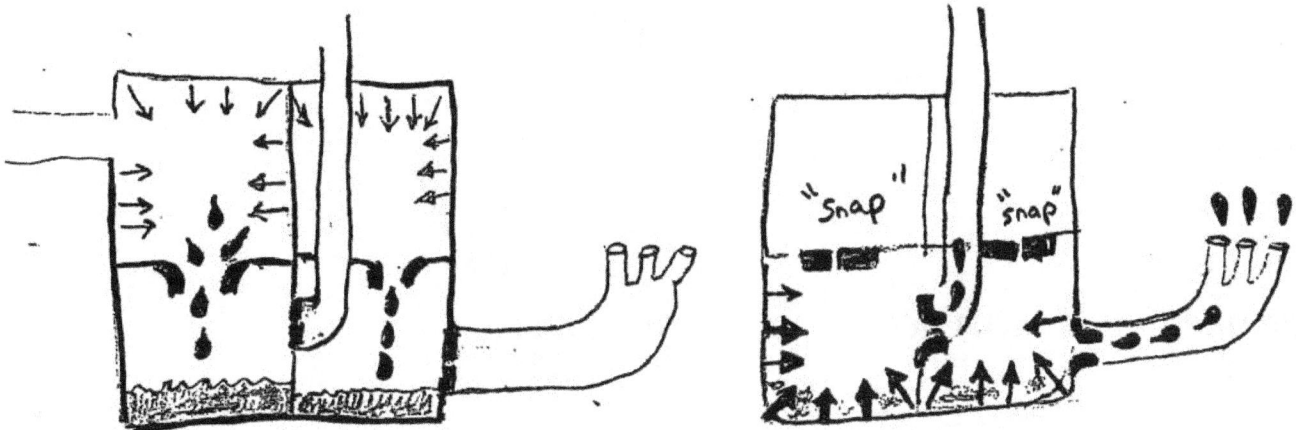

"Dub" End of Systole: the blood has been pushed through the pulmonic valve and aorta, the ventricles have relaxed, the pulmonic aand aortic valves snap shut. S2

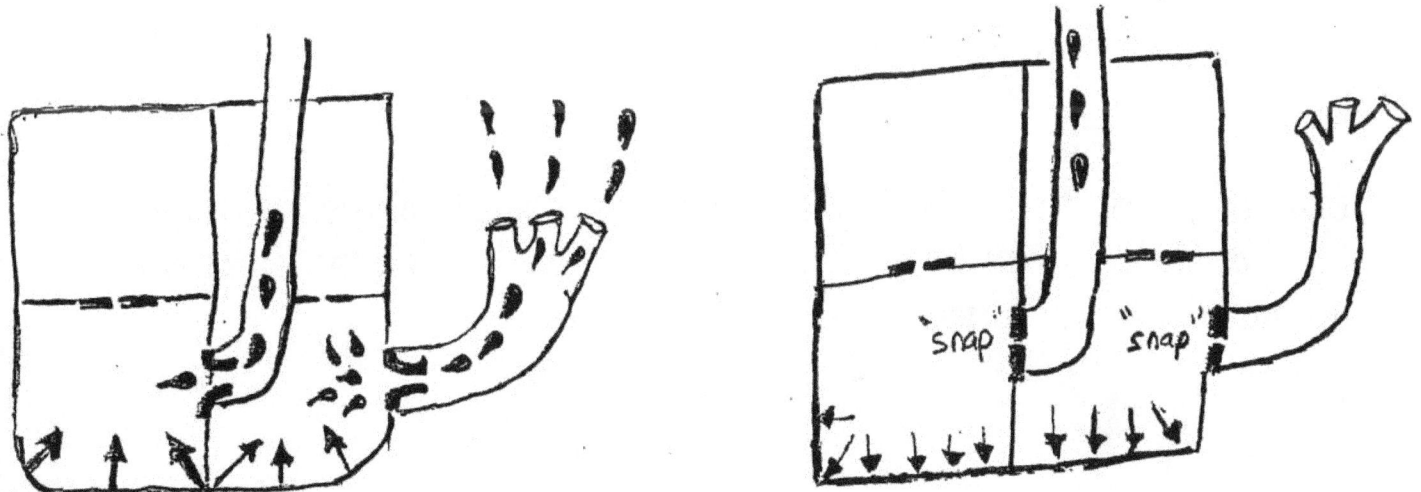

ABNORMAL HEART SOUNDS

Murmurs – there are two types.

Stenosis If any of the four valves are to stiff to open completely the blood flowing through makes a sound (murmur). To get an idea of what you are hearing, let's look at a water balloon.

If water flows out of a water balloon unrestricted, there is no noise.

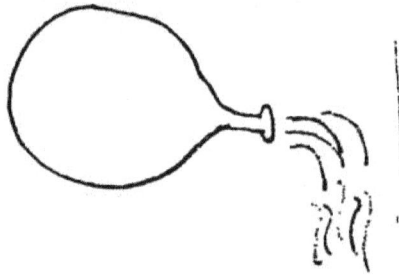

If the opening is restricted it will make a noise.

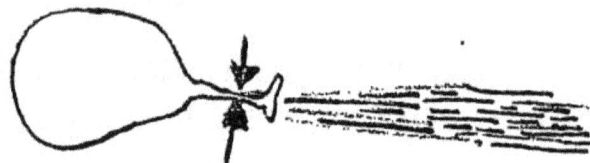

Similarly blood flows easily through normal heart valves. If the valves are stiff they do not open fully. The blood rushes through the narrowed orifice and makes a lot of noise.

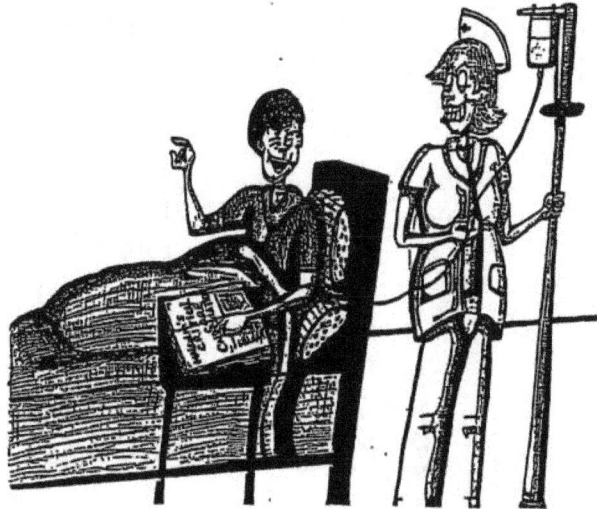
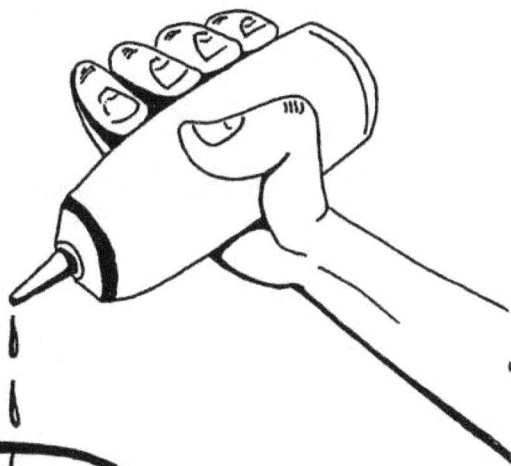
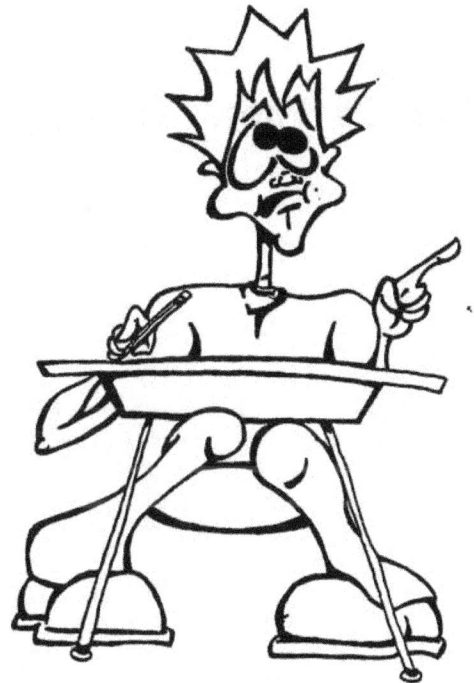

Murmurs the second type

The other source of murmurs is incompetent or leaky valves. Incompetant valves do not close with a tight seal.

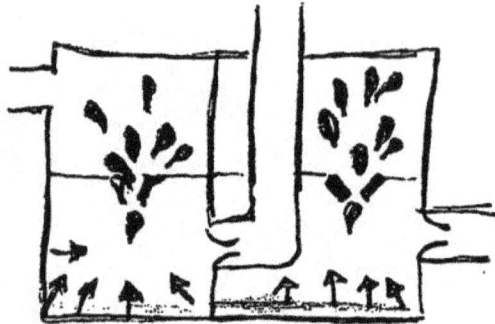

If the valves don't close properly blood leaks backward. In this picture blood is leaking backward through the mitral and tricuspid valve during systole (i.e. from the ventricles toward the atria). This "regurgitant" murmur sounds like a blowing sound, but could sound like a honk or a sea gull cry.

We now know murmurs. The next question is, "When do they occur?"

DIASTOLIC or SYSTOLIC HEART SOUNDS
How do we figure that out?

systolic?

"Lub" the first heart sound is the start of ventricular systole. It is the start of ventricular systole, the closure of mitral and tricuspid valves due to ventricular contraction. Any sounds that occur after the first heart sound are "systolic". S1 is lower in pitch and lasts longer. A pulse at the carotid artery will be felt at the same time S1 is heard. The heart sound following the longer pause is S1 (Diastole is 2/3 of the time elapsed in a heart beat).

diastolic?

"Dub" The second heart sound caused by closure of the aortic and pulmonic valves is the start of diastole. That makes sense. Diastole happens after the ventricles have squeezed out the blood. Diastole is longer than systole. The heart sound following the longer pause is S1 and the other one… well…that is S2.

Determining S1 and S2 will be important in identifying abnormal heart sounds.

now we will learn about…

DIASTOLIC MURMURS

After the ventricles have squeezed blood through the whole body and lungs the pressure drops in the ventricles, the aortic and pulmonic valves snap shut, S2, "Dub". Then it starts all over again. The atria start to drop blood into the ventricles. In other words: diastole.

If any heart sounds are heart sounds are heard during diastole, they are called diastolic murmurs.

Lets say due to an incompetent aortic valve blood leaked back (regurgitant) into the left ventricle. That would occur after S2 and would be called diastolic.

Said one more time pulmonic or aortic regurgitation due to insufficient valves would be a diastolic murmur

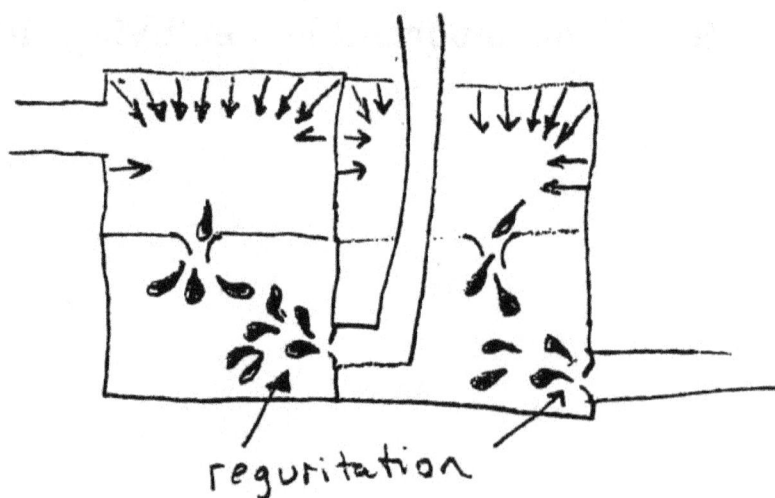

reguritation

more...

DIASTOLIC MURMURS

Mitral or tricuspid stenosis cause high blood flow rates through the constricted valves.

You would hear this noise after the "Dub". It is a diastolic murmur.

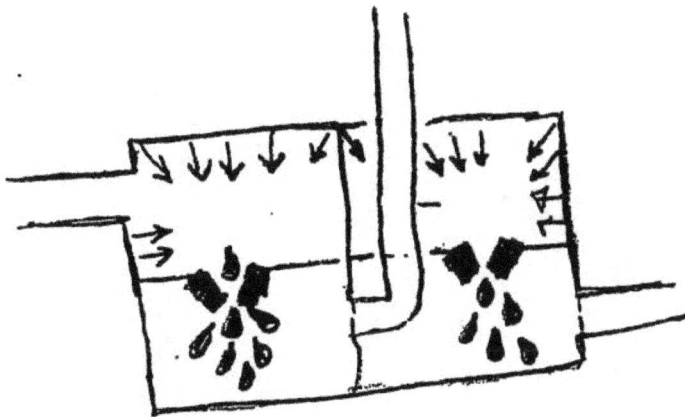

There are....

FOUR DIASTOLIC MURMURS

AORTIC REGURGITATION
PULMONIC REGURGITATION
MITRAL STENOSIS
TRICUSPID STENOSIS

Now what?

SYSTOLIC MURMURS

After "Lub", it's systole when the blood is being squeezed out of the ventricles. If the aortic or pulmonic valve is stenotic, it is stiff and doesn't open completely. The blood is forced through a small opening which causes fast turbulent flow. The noisy flow which occurs after S1 is a systolic murmur.

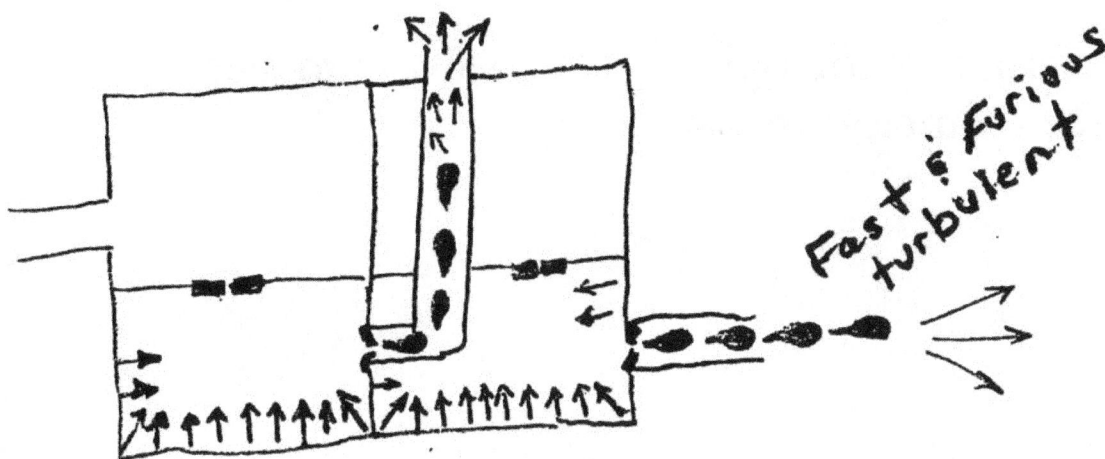

Fast & Furious turbulent

After stenotic systolic murmurs.....

REGURGITANT SYSTOLIC MURMURS

The ventricles contract and squeeze blood out."Lub". S1 The mitral and tricuspid valve snap shut.

If either of the valves does not close tight and blood leaks backward, a murmur can be heard before the end of systole (S2, "Dub")

For that reason insufficient tricuspid or mitral valves produce systolic murmurs while the ventricles are contracting.

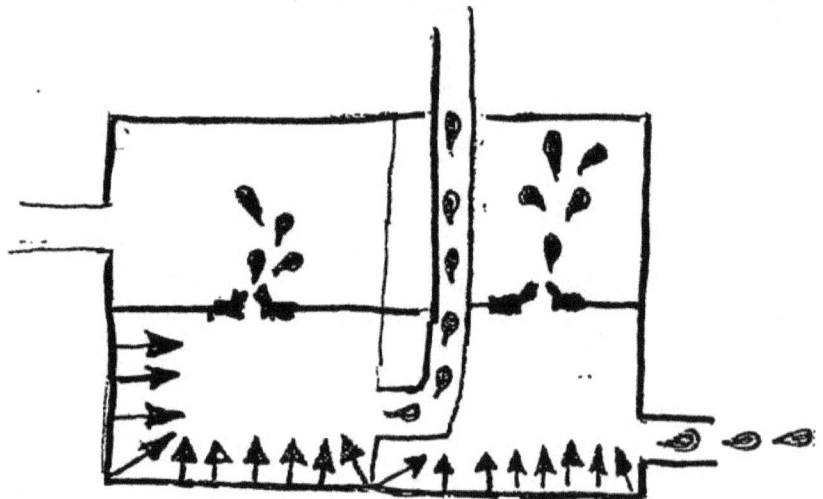

There are....
FOUR SYSTOLIC MURMURS

mitral regurgitation

tricuspid regurgitatiom

aortic stenosis

pulmonic stenosis

No more murmurs…
S2 PHYSIOLOGIC SPLIT

When ventricular systole ends, the aortic valve normally closes before the pulmonic valve. During expiration (when you breath not when you die), the interval is so small, the sounds are heard as one "Dub".

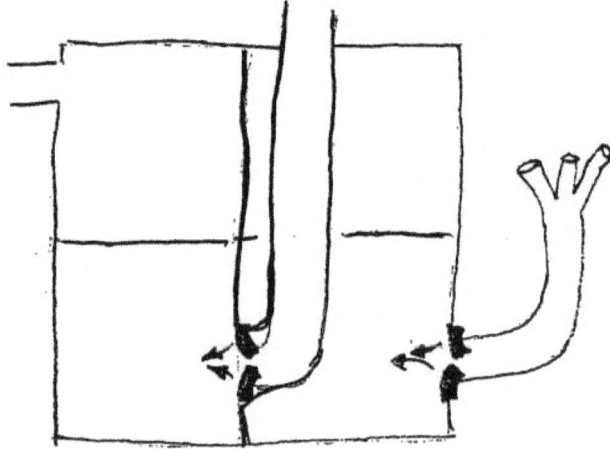

Inspiration is the lungs expanding and drawing in air. You know that. The biggest (but not only) cause of this is the diaphragm muscle lowering. This expands the entire chest contents. The whole box enclosed by the ribs gets bigger. What matters for us is that more room allows the vena cava to expand and allow more blood flow. So, during inspiration (breathing, not artistic) venous return to the right ventricle increases - which prolongs right ventricle systole. That makes sense. More blood takes longer to squeeze out. So the pulmonic closure is delayed. That is called a split. A split is normal.

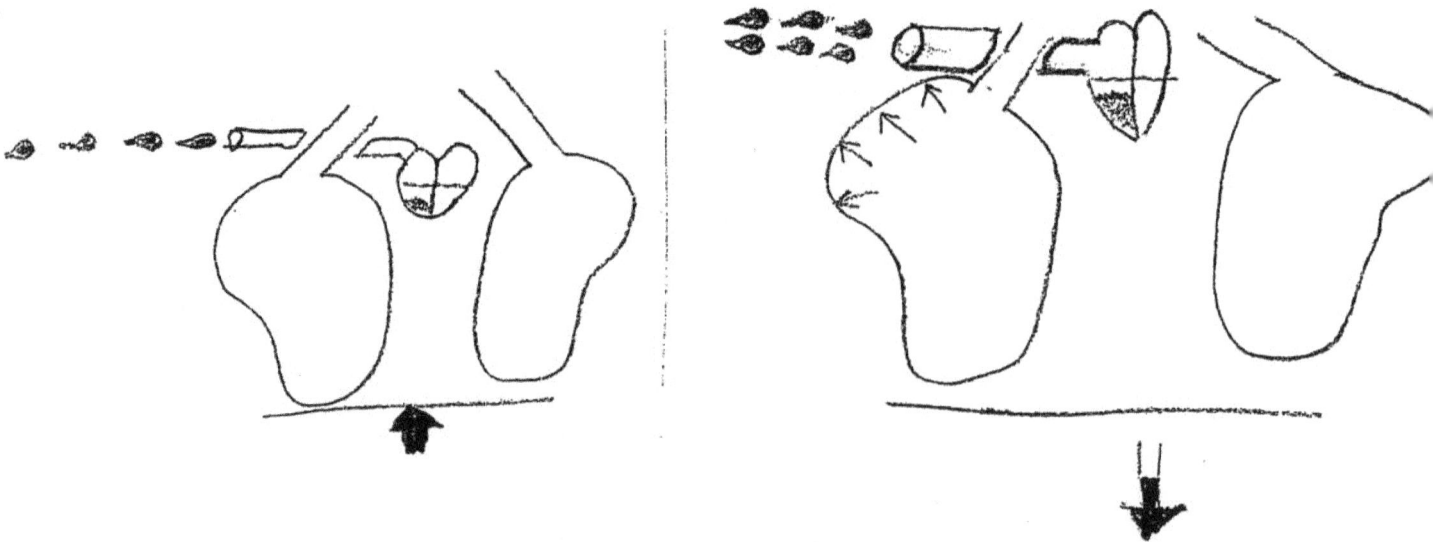

S3   and   S4

S3 and S4 are two abnormal sounds heard during diastole, after S2 and before S1. They are not related to valve closure.

S₃

S3 is caused by rapid early filling of a noncompliant ventricle in early diastole. It occurs shortly after atrial contraction, or shortly after S2. It is an early sigh of CHF. Because the ventricle walls are stiff they do not empty as much blood as a more compliant ventricle.

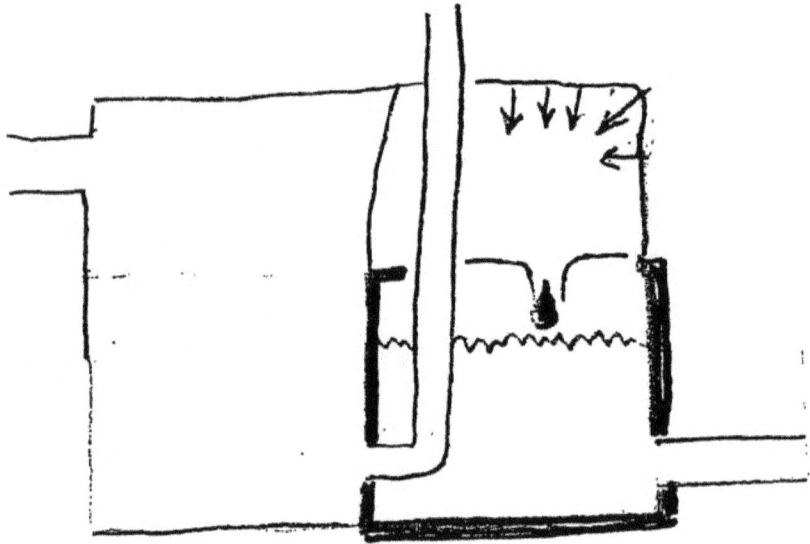

S₄

S4 occurs later in diastole than S3. In other words it is closer to S1. S4 is caused by atrial contractions trying to fill an already mostly filled stiff noncompliant ventricle.

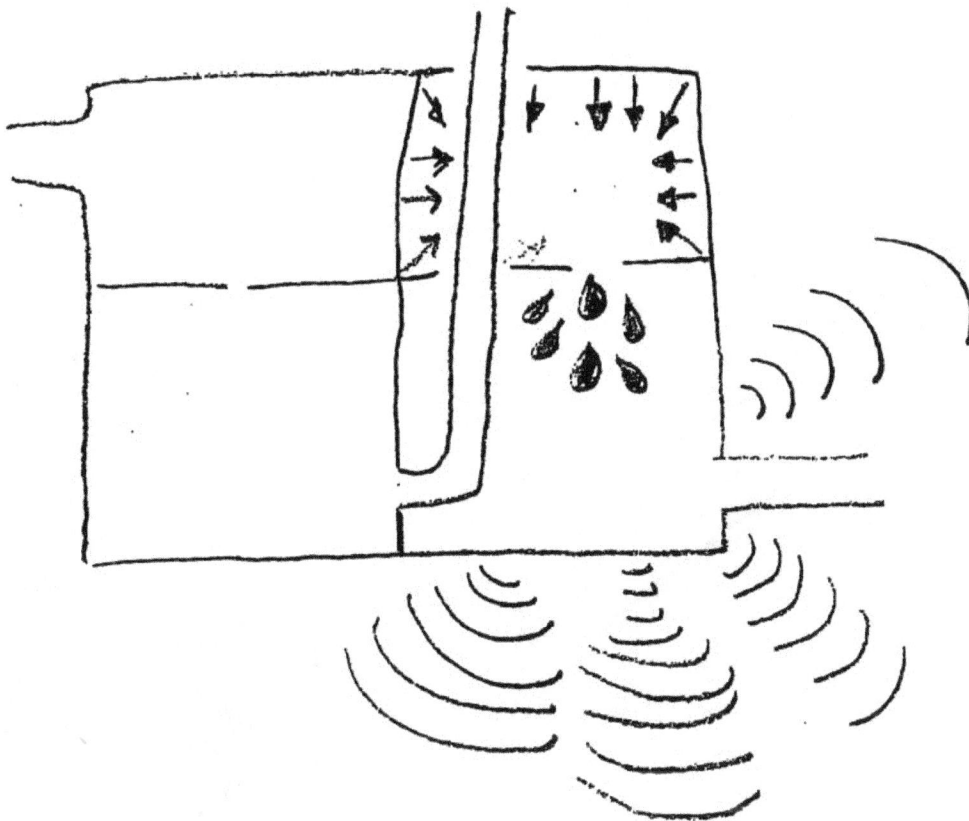

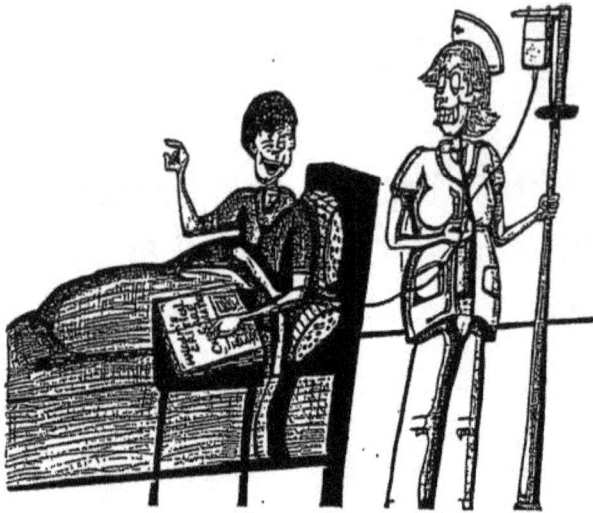
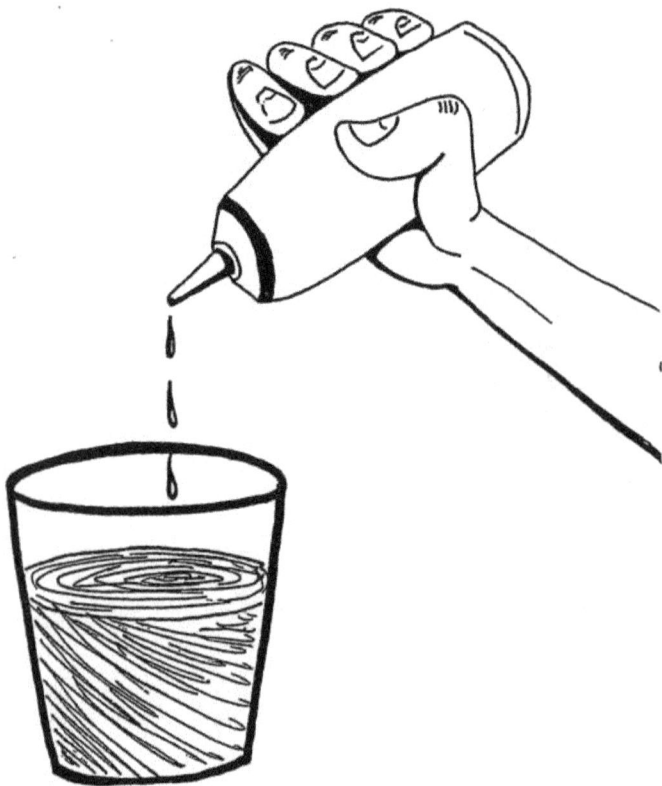
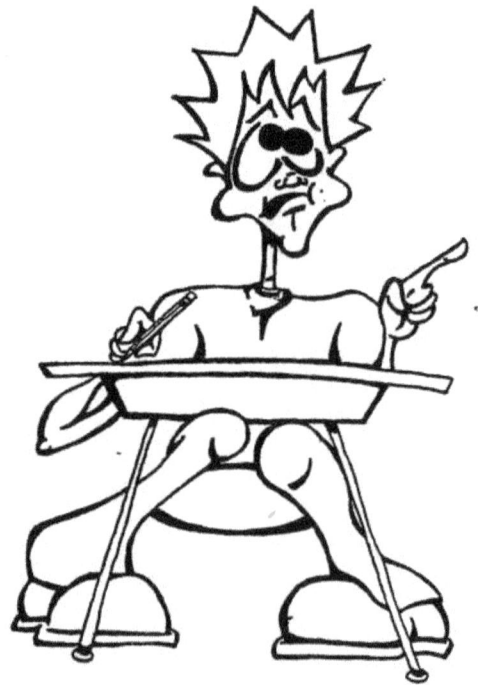

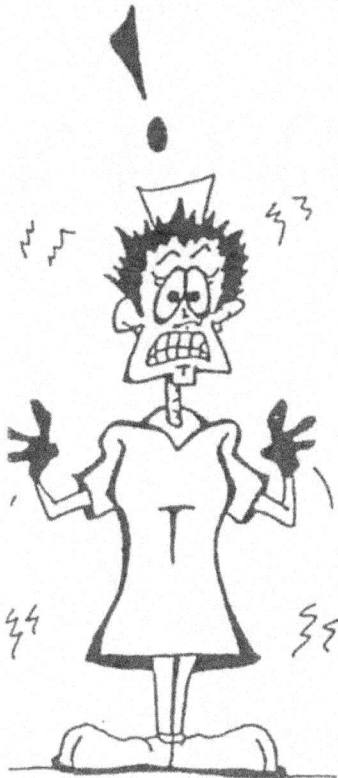
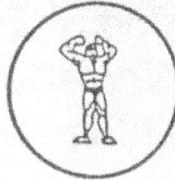
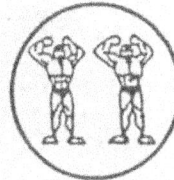
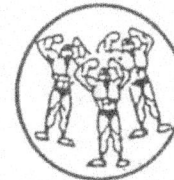
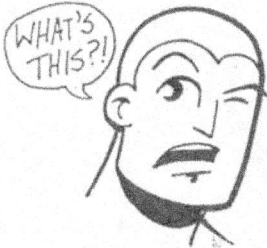 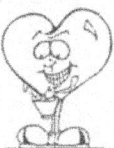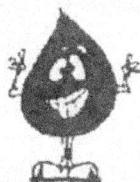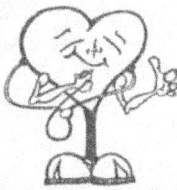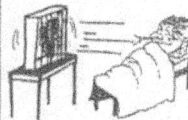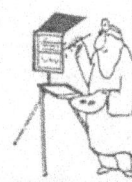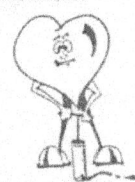

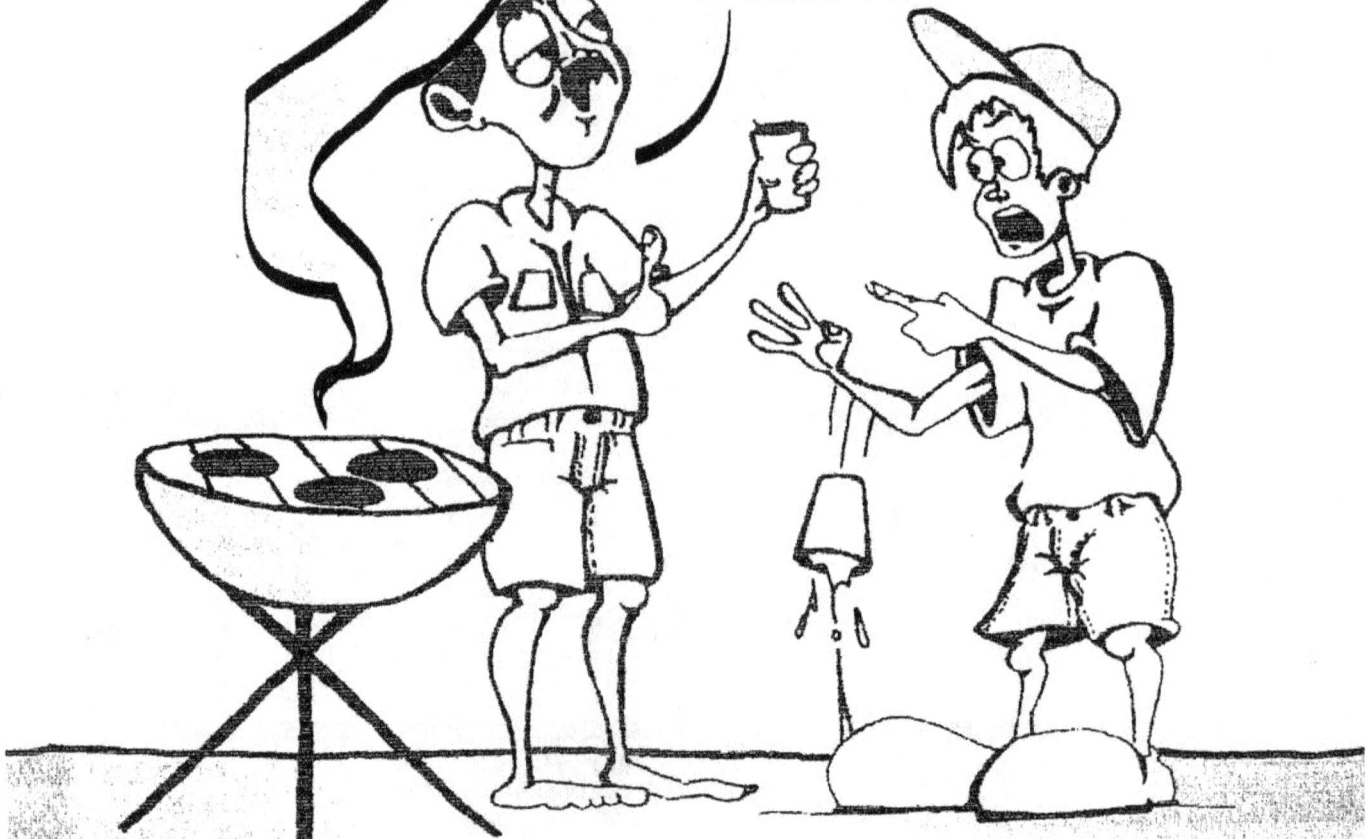

Simplified Heart Sounds ©2005

Retail: $7.95

ISBN 0-9725483-5-1

9780972548359

0 700814 498047

7 00814 49804 7

www.ingramcontent.com/pod-product-compliance
Lightning Source LLC
Chambersburg PA
CBHW051341200326
41520CB00033B/7437